FULL CIRCLE

Esther,
Let me share a part
of my "family" with you
through this book and
say "thanks" for all your
support and love and
friendship.   Love and peace,
                        Pat

Judy is my cousin —
writing about my great-aunt,
her mother.

FULL CIRCLE

Experiences with an Aging Parent

Judith Lee-Hoffer

illustrated by Carolyn Shugar

Detselig Enterprises Ltd.

Canadian Cataloguing in Publication Data

Lee-Hoffer, Judith, 1939-
Full circle

ISBN 1-55059-042-1

1. Aging parents—Canada—Family relationships.
2. Adult children—Canada—Family relationships.
3. Lee-Hoffer, Judith, 1939-   I. Title.
HQ1064.C2L43 1992   306.874   C92-091334-2

Detselig Enterprises Ltd.
Suite 210, 1220 Kensington Rd. N.W.
Calgary, Alberta
T2N 3P5

Detselig Enterprises Ltd. appreciates the financial assistance for its 1992 publishing program from Canada Council and Alberta Foundation for the Arts.

Printed in Canada   SAN 115-0324   ISBN 1-55059-042-1

To my mother who exemplifies that our ordinary lives can make a difference

Contents

A c k n o w l e d g m e n t s

I truly feel blessed by God and grateful to everyone who has contributed to my life—relatives, friends, teachers, clients, neighbors, colleagues, even pets. However, space permits me to acknowledge only those who have been most influential in the creation of this book.

My loving and lovable partner Art who encourages me to be my own person and supports me in pursuing my dreams.

My son Aaron who, as a child, taught me to appreciate dinosaurs, whales, eagles, and sunflowers and today still challenges me to expand my thinking.

My daughter Naomi, close to my heart, a beautiful combination of strength and gentleness who fills me with hope for the women of the future.

My mother-in-law Rose Hoffer, an inspiring, independent eighty-nine-year-old who is a prolific painter and active volunteer at a hospital and a synagogue.

The warm memories of my father Ole Lee, sister Eleanor, and brothers Douglas, Lloyd, Raymond and Milton who all shared my love for Mom.

My courageous, nurturing sisters-in-law Muriel, Helen and Bernice who continue to grow more dear to me.

Nieces and nephews who also make their unique contributions to the loving fabric of our family.

The staff and members of St. David's United Church who took a personal interest in my mother and who have been most receptive to our stories.

Kathleen Gleeson, whose extensive vocabulary is matched by her generous heart.

Jack Heynen, Helen Hooker, Mickey Markert, Mike McIntyre and Moira Nasim, long-time-interested and supportive friends.

Compassionate confidante, Penny Goodson who, across the miles, has always cheered me on in my endeavors.

Yvonne Fries and Eveline Wheatley Goodall, my "full moon cohorts" who have never wavered in their faith in me and my writing aspirations.

Marge Robinson, congruent friend and kindred spirit who respected my designated writing times and thus taught me to do the same.

My valued and affirming friend Stan Errett who was the first to read my vignettes and encourage me to seek publication.

John Griffith and Helen Sanderson who invited me to read some vignettes in public; and Muriel Duncan who first risked their publication and urged me to write more.

Dear and creative friend, Beth Hemstreet who first referred to me as "a writer."

The many thoughtful people who telephoned or wrote to express their appreciation of my stories.

My personable, enthusiastic and committed typist Michelle Burgess.

Talented and perceptive Carolyn Shugar, who has captured and portrayed the essence of my vignettes in her delightful drawings.

Leslie Chapman, my gentle and clear-thinking editor, with whom it has been a pleasure to work.

Thank you.

Introduction

Life is a fascinating and challenging endeavor. Wherever we are on the continuum between birth and death, we must frequently make decisions as to where to focus our attention and how best to expend our energy. Despite the uncontrollable aspects of our existence, we cannot escape the responsibility for our choices. The choices we make determine the direction of our lives.

When I am confronted by myriad expectations and opportunities, I need to stop and ask myself, "What choice will be most meaning full?" Occasionally the answer which emerges from within is not what I prefer to hear. So in my attempt to drown out this quiet voice, I become even busier pursuing less important goals. However, no matter what I do, my inner sense of knowing prevails. When I finally choose to acknowledge and act on this intuitive guidance, I experience a sense of rightness, of self-fulfillment. It is with such a sense this book has been written.

Despite our countless differences, one universal experience we share with all humanity is that we are born of parents. While the global population is annually increasing by 1.7 percent, the number of elderly is increasing by 2.4 percent. Naturally, increased longevity will mean a longer duration of family relationships. In our North American society, the majority of parents and children will share fifty years of their lifetime. By the same token, most grandchildren will have the opportunity to interact for at least twenty years with their grandparents.

The vignettes in this book reflect my personal experiences. In no way are they meant to imply, "this is how elder care ought to be given." Indeed, in our Western society, where such a high value is placed on self-sufficiency, most elders favor a lifestyle which permits them to live as independently as possible. Many older people—some aided by practical community services and emotional support from their families—are well able to cope successfully in their own homes. Others prefer to relocate in senior citizen communities or move into lodges where they maintain some privacy while still free to enjoy the company of others.

Elder self-esteem is greatly enhanced by involvement in formal organizations and participation in satisfying group activities. Therefore being cloistered, safe, secure and loved in an adult child's home, as my mother was, does not necessarily ensure a desirable quality of life.

Recent studies do indicate, however, that regardless of where aging parents reside, their well-being is strongly influenced by the amount of affection and communication they experience in their relationships with their children near or far. They also highly value and benefit from their ability to reciprocate the help given to them. In fact, the overall aid given by older parents to their adult children at least equals and sometimes surpasses the amount received.

It has been estimated at least twenty percent of the Canadian population will eventually require institutionalization due to age and declining health. My knowledge of such facilities was minimal until I began searching for respite care. Only then did I discover that some of the nursing homes available were more pleasant and provided more services than I had imagined. Unfortunately, by that time Mom was no longer able to articulate her perceptions or concerns when touring these places.

My experience made me realize how helpful it would be for parents and children to become knowledgeable about available resources and alternative living arrangements before actually requiring them. Such information could dissipate archaic fears and facilitate more rational decisions. Also, early enquiries would heighten awareness regarding gaps in the diversity and flexibility of needed services and conditions which demand improvement. It is easier to be empowered advocates while not yet dependent upon what is available.

In some situations the wisest, most desirable choice for everyone concerned may be to form a multi-generational household. Surprisingly enough, an American study predicts twenty-five percent of couples in the thirty to fifty year range will do so. Certainly both young and old need to be involved in such a decision since there will be implications for everyone. It is important to recognize each person's physical and emotional boundaries and discuss how these will be respected. Agreements need to be made as to what people can realistically expect of each other. Each family will have its unique concerns. Does Grandpa do his own cooking? At what volume can Granddaughter play her rock music? Are outside babysitters still to be hired when Grandma is at home? Where can one leave personal belongings undisturbed in a disordered state? Families are dynamic. If open, honest communication is maintained between members it is more likely the meeting of each person's changing needs will be successfully negotiated.

My mother was forty-five when I, the youngest of eight siblings by eleven years, was born. After my father's death when I was seven, Mom and I lived alone together for nine years. My only sister, sixteen years older, provided a link for me to the modern world. At times of crisis she would return home and look after us. She died when I was twenty-four.

Mom was a nurturer who unconditionally loved all children. Seldom did she tell me what to do. "You know what's best," was her admonition when I was faced with a difficult decision. She spanked me only once and told me later how much she regretted ever resorting to such behavior. In one of our home movies taken after our first child was born, Mom is standing by quietly and supportively holding the safety pins while I awkwardly struggle to bathe and diaper our infant. After Mom came to live with our family, she convinced us washing our dishes and mending our clothes gave her tremendous pleasure. She was also very sensitive to our needs for some privacy and seemed to know just when to quietly retreat to her own place. Fortunately, I was married to a generous man, secure enough in himself not to desire my constant attention, who welcomed Mom into our home.

I'm giving you this background to help you better understand what partially contributed to our family's ability to provide the care Mom required in her latter years. Years when, although not formally diagnosed, she undoubtedly suffered from Alzheimer's disease. Had we not had the family history we did, I am not certain our living arrangement would have worked. If my childhood experience had been one of mistreatment, I could have easily stored up a lot of resentment. Under the stress of caregiving, this pent-up anger might have been expressed by repeating what had been done to me.

Contrary to popular belief, the reported cases of elder abuse usually occur in situations where a partially incapacitated spouse or adult child acts abusively toward the aged person upon whom he or she is dependent. Little is actually known of abuse by caregivers of the elderly. Since we have only recently become more aware of the extent to which women and children are subject to abuse, I wonder if elder abuse still remains largely hidden. Certainly there is potential for such abuse. The frail elderly are extremely vulnerable. Unlike children who will eventually grow up and be able "to tell," the aged person's power will continue to diminish. Undoubtedly, the vast majority of caregivers, employed or related, have no intention of acting abusively. Such abuse would be most likely to occur only under the heavy, if not impossible demands of the role coupled with lack of appreciation and support. Indeed, caregivers must be on the receiving end of nurturing as well if they are to provide the high quality of compassionate care intended.

I do believe at our core we are all good people. Everything considered, each one of us has done the very best we can at any given moment in time. This doesn't mean we don't all, including our parents, make some mistakes despite our good intentions. Unfortunately, some of you may have been hurt a great deal by your parents. If so, you need to give yourself opportunities to heal from those hurts and reconcile with your past. One of the most loving things to do may be to acknowledge you and your parents need some distance apart. Professional caregivers, unencumbered by shared history, may be better able to provide your parents with quality care. You will then be free to consciously use your contacts with your parents to come to terms with your past and create the best possible relationship in the present. Given the opportunity, aging parents are often eager to make amends. Old or young, it is crucial to our well-being to become realistic and accepting of each other's limitations. At the same time, we must never lose sight of the potential for positive change in all our relationships.

Researchers have exploded the myth that we in our modern society abandon our elderly. On the contrary, estimates are eighty percent of the long-term care required by older persons is provided by family and friends.

The term "sandwich generation" has been coined to describe people who are squeezed between parenting their children and caretaking their aging parents. As our life span lengthens, this generation is becoming increasingly older. Presently the average age of such caregivers is fifty-seven; an age at which they may well be involved in their own mid-life transition. If so, they will be dealing concurrently with a number of important issues: children leaving or remaining at home for economic reasons; the prospect of losing their parents; and a heightened awareness of their own mortality.

Regrettably, even in this day and age, the major burdens and satisfactions of caregiving are still expected of and assumed by women. While men may assist financially, research findings indicate seventy-eight percent of parental care is provided by women. In her writings, Rita Robinson suggests that on the average a woman will spend eighteen years of her life assisting an elderly parent. Those who encounter most stress are those daughters living alone with an ill parent.

Nowadays many women are gainfully employed outside their homes. To furnish the necessary care for elderly parents many will either jeopardize their careers by quitting or taking leaves of absence or will become emotionally and physically exhausted by attempting to do it all. This is particularly true of women in the lower economic group who cannot afford to enlist the services of others. Reluctant to risk interruptions during working hours because of financial considerations, their leisure time is converted into caregiving.

Hopefully, in time, our consciousness will be raised. Just as we are now recognizing the benefits of fathers taking a more active role in parenting, so will we eventually realize all lives will be enriched when there is more equitable participation in the care of the aged. Indeed, it will be the forward-thinking industries and governments which will prudently begin making necessary provisions to allow both male and female employees to meet the needs of elderly parents.

When my mother first came to live with our family, I assumed the responsibility of ensuring no one was inconvenienced by this arrangement. After all, she was *my* mother, I rationalized. I attempted to act as a buffer between her, my husband and children. In time I grew emotionally weary and had to abandon this role. When I did everyone benefited. Yes, there were occasional conflicts, but, more significantly, genuine caring relationships had more of an opportunity to develop.

In the earlier years, Mom's presence in our home provided a stability for the children which allowed me the emotional freedom to pursue some of my learning and professional goals. However, later, as Mom became more frail and required more care, I found even coping with part-time employment stressful. The unpredictability of the care required and the need for constant vigilance took its toll. Community services such as Meals On Wheels and Home Care relieved some of the burden. Home visits from church volunteers and friends brought some of the outside world to Mom. Subsidized taxi service and an afternoon of tea and conversation for shut-ins at a local senior citizens' lodge encouraged her to venture out.

Sibling relationships become increasingly important as we grow older. There can be a special bonding with those who have shared our roots. As aging parents require care, either sibling rivalries rekindle or a closer co-operative relationship develops among the adult children. Fortunately for me, Mom was loved and wanted by all my family. Across the miles they phoned and wrote. When Mom was no longer able to travel, occasionally one of them would come and stay with her so we could take a vacation. Our relatives' ability to refrain from criticism and their expression of support and appreciation for the care we gave Mom made a tremendous difference to me.

Friends, counsellors, and self-help groups can help reduce strain and be an invaluable source of support. We, in the middle generation, have been taught to respect our parents. We may feel guilty if we complain about them. Often we view ourselves as incompetent and unable to reciprocate the quality of care we received from them as children. According to some studies, one of the most stressful aspects of our role may reside in attempts to protect our parents from becoming aware of their diminishing capabilities. As we lose the kinkeeper, the comforter, the parental companion of yesteryears, we may enter a chronic state of grief. Therefore, for our own emotional health, we need safe places with understanding people to whom we can vent our frustrations, fears and sadness. Doing so will reduce the strain and will enable us to maintain our caregiving role in a more loving way. Aging parents, too, need other people who will not regard them as ungrateful when they voice their frustrations in coping with the younger generations. Elders also benefit from an empathic listener with whom they can discuss the irrevocable losses of time, abilities and loved ones they experience in their advancing years.

We, in our society, have grown up in a mechanistic age. Youth and productivity are valued. Encouraged to focus on our "doing," it is easy to forget we are truly human "beings." We can easily lose touch with our uniqueness. Instead, the tendency is to treat ourselves and each other like machines which come off an assembly line; replaceable machines easily discarded when they break down or become obsolete. No wonder death terrifies us and we work desperately hard at denying the inevitable changes of aging. We prefer the smoothness of youth to the interesting lines of experience. Perhaps we often avoid contact with the elderly because they confront us with some of the impending realities of our future.

How crucial for all of humanity that we begin to alter our mechanistic viewpoint! We need to realize that each of us, distinguishable by a mere thumbprint, is unique and definitely irreplaceable. Creator of our personal story in this life, each of us makes and leaves our indelible mark. Unlike machines, we human beings continue to develop, to unfold throughout our lifetime. We benefit when we learn to welcome and accept our naturally evolving cycles.

Death is truly the definer of life and we must learn how to embrace it as such. We do not know for certain what follows this gift of life. Yet, few of us can honestly gaze into the universe and not be convinced this earthly life is but a minute part of what there is to know. Perhaps it will become possible to echo the words of Dag Hammarskjold, "For all that has been, thanks! For all that will be, yes!"

No matter what our past relationship has been like, perhaps each of us would benefit by spending some time alone with our parents in their advancing years. An opportunity to reconcile; to express regrets and appreciations; and to discover the unique beauty in our aged parent. Maybe in discerning that beauty we will grow less fearful of our own aging.

I feel very privileged to have had the opportunity to spend as much time as I did with my mother. Each day, no matter what occurred, offered its own gifts. I hope you will enjoy reading about our experiences together. Most of all, I hope you will be inspired to become even more aware of the delights, sometimes hidden yet always present, in the everydayness of your own important life.

Background and statistical information for the introduction was primarily gleaned from the following books and journals.

Abel, Emily. *Love Is Not Enough: Family Care of the Frail Elderly*. Washington, D.C.: American Public Health Association, 1987.

Bumagin, Victoria and Hirn, Kathryn. *Aging Is A Family Affair.* New York: Thomas Y. Crowell Publisher, 1979.

Canadian Journal on Aging. Ottawa: Canadian Association on Gerentology.

Connides, Ingrid. *Family Ties and Aging*. Markham, Ontario: Butterworth and Company Ltd., 1989.

Levin, Norma Jean. *How to Care for Your Parents: A Handbook for Adult Children*. Washington, D.C.: Storm King Press, 1987.

Jorvik, Lessy and Small, Gary. *Parentcare. A Commonsense Guide for Adult Children*. New York: Crown Publishers Inc., 1988.

Robinson, Rita. *When Your Parents Need You*. Santa Monica, CA: IBS Press, 1990.

The Gerentologist. Washington: Gerentological Society.

Beginnings

In 1906, at the age of twelve, Mom immigrated to Canada, leaving behind on the Minnesota prairies, her parents, eight sisters and two brothers. Secretly promised a dime if she didn't cry, she managed without a tear to say good-bye to each one until she came to her own dear "Mama." Then the flood gates opened.

She had decided on this venture because she liked excitement and because she felt sorry for her older sister, *my grandmother* Gunda. Gunda was the young bride of a new minister, *grandfather* who had been called to serve as a pastor in rural Manitoba. Mom anticipated how lonely her sister would be so far from her family. Therefore, with little persuasion she agreed to accompany them north.

In the years following, during bitter winters, baptisms, fowl suppers, funerals and long sermons, Mom became acquainted with the pressures and rewards of ministerial life. This appreciation and empathy for pastors and their families continued into adulthood. From farm to town to city the church has remained a focal point in her life.

Fortunately, in our large urban church, our minister has sensed his importance to Mom. Even with hundreds of families requesting attention he has made time for the occasional visit. What a gift! Mom's whole world has been brightened by his coming.

"You know, the Reverend took and held my hands while we prayed today," Mom confides to me, her aged face glowing with appreciation.

Attending church on Sunday is still the highlight of her week. Almost without fail, once we're settled in our seats, Mom draws my attention to the front of the sanctuary. "Look who's there!," she whispers. She smiles and nods. I smile, too, certain there's not another member of the congregation present who's as pleased or surprised as Mom to discover our minister leading the worship!

❋　　❋　　❋

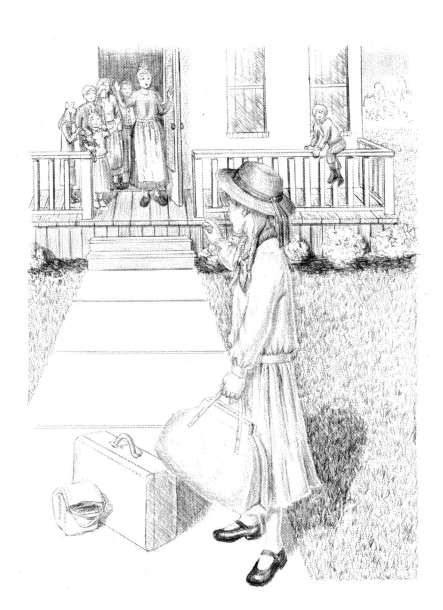

A Blessing

After years of renting accommodations, my husband and I finally were financially ready to contemplate the purchase of our first home. It was Mom who suggested, and we agreed, that when the actual possession date arrived she would move into a senior citizen's lodge. With such a plan in mind we still included her in our house hunting. Frequently on these excursions, as we were being shown around by the real estate agent, Mom's voice would beckon us to some remote corner of the basement. "You know, I'm just thinking I could be quite comfortable with a spot here. Wouldn't take much fixing up at all. Then you could have part of my pension cheque to help with the mortgage payments."

We heard the message. Without making any promises, we began searching for a home with Mom in mind. Unfortunately most affordable houses offered only standard-sized bedrooms with small windows. We could not visualize Mom cooped up in one of these nor our whole family able to function well in such close proximity.

Eventually, it was a private newspaper ad which caught our attention. Further investigation revealed an attractive, cozy home boasting a fire place and an open-beam cedar ceiling; situated across from a play park; and within walking distance from a church as well as from the university where my husband taught. And, believe it or not, this house also had an adjacent car port renovated into a large family room with lots of windows and a private entrance—an ideal environment for Mom. Indeed, the place seemed perfectly suited to all our needs. Without hesitation we signed the contract.

Days later unexpected financial complications arose and we found ourselves short one thousand dollars for the down payment. I cried as my husband phoned to explain and regretfully decline the purchase. Within hours the owners called back saying that, despite the fact they had several other prospective buyers, they had decided they preferred us to have their home, consequently they were willing to reduce the price accordingly. What joy!

Even today, fifteen years later, as I see the afternoon sun streaming in through Mom's windows, I know this is where we are meant to live. Within these walls we are truly blessed.

✳   ✳   ✳

P r o m i s e s

Some slick executive in the credit office of an immense corporate department store received a personal phone call this morning. It was from Mom, explaining with simple honesty why her monthly ten dollar payment would arrive later than usual.

I hope that busy executive was as touched as I was by the naive belief that in this impersonal multi-billion dollar business world, an individual and her ten dollars still count.

*　*　*

L i f e ' s   L e s s o n s

I'll never forget dear Mrs. Paulson," Mom reminisced, "especially the day she came over to see me on the homestead. I was feeling so blue. We had just buried our infant; the little girl I had wanted so much. Through my tears I said to Mrs. Paulson, 'But I wanted her to live!' Instead of giving me the sympathy I had anticipated, she admonished, 'Well Clara, we can't always have what we want.' I was rather taken aback at the time but actually that was good for me to hear. It helped me to dry my eyes and get on with living."

Occasionally, Mom repeated the admonition to me during my growing-up years. I re-interpreted it to mean, "It's all right to want it all. However, if you don't get what you want, don't waste time feeling sorry for yourself." I, in turn, would teach my children, "It's important to ask for what you want. There's nothing wrong in asking. You also have the right to sometimes say no when asked."

One afternoon my five-year-old daughter was busy drawing a picture while Mom and I talked. Leaning over her shoulder, Mom suggested it might be a good idea to add a particular animal to her drawing. My daughter ignored her, intent upon her own creation. Mom persisted, repeating her suggestion. Still no response. Mom was beginning her third intervention when my daughter finally stopped her coloring, looked directly up to her grandmother and with gentle firmness reminded her. "You can't have everything you want, you know Nana."

Forty-five years and two generations later, Mom smiled and said nothing.

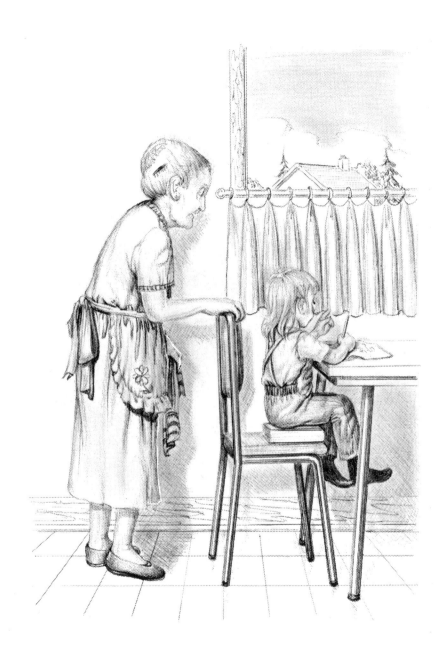

G r o c e r y   L i s t

Most grocery lists are uninteresting columns, denoting quantities of items. Not Mom's. Forgetting some of the brand names, her orders become colorful descriptions of what she wants purchased as well as what she does not need. I found this old one in my jacket pocket today:

> *A package of those tasty cookies—the ones with the white filling—my company liked them.*
>
> *Stafford needs some soft food—the harder kind hurts his teeth—his mouth seems to be getting worse.*
>
> *I don't need any of the yellow stuff you put on bread.*
>
> *Thank you. I'll make this right with you!*

*   *   *

Our Treasure

Life was hectic with two children fifteen months apart. Always some need to be met, some little person demanding attention.

Like a calm storm, Mom was there ready to lend a hand. Often she washed the dishes; always she mended our clothes. She seemed to assume these tasks almost eagerly, without complaint. I, indeed, was grateful for her help. Engaged in varied activities with the children, I'd occasionally comment, "My, Nana's such a treasure!"

Even with Mom's support, full-time motherhood did not prove to be the dream I had anticipated. One day after throwing a piece of Tupperware across the kitchen in frustration, I realized I must make some changes in my lifestyle. I decided to return to part-time employment outside the home. I was confident with more space of my own, I would become a better mother.

We were fortunate to eventually find a loving, competent babysitter. However, in our children's changing world it was Mom who provided them with emotional security. Without interfering, she was there to offer a knee to sit on, a listening ear, an extra hug whenever needed.

One day, upon returning from work, our babysitter greeted me, eager to share her story. While playing that afternoon, our daughter had confided to her, "You know, Nana's Mommy's treasure and when I grow up Mommy's going to be my treasure too."

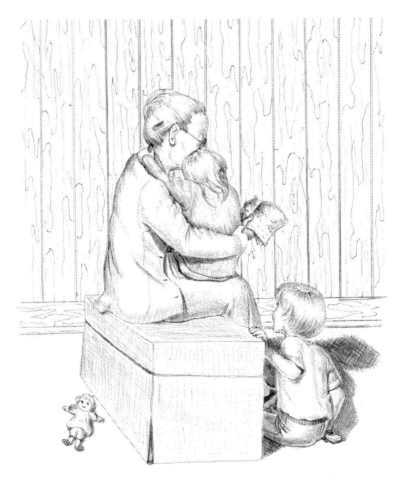

Anticipation

Mom's done it again! I see it through the window. She's raised the mailbox lid in preparation for the postman's delivery. It's as if she believes this open receptacle will have the power to beckon a much awaited letter from a loved one.

I hope it does.

* * *

The Blanket

From the time I was a small child, whenever I laid down for a rest, Mom, without fail, would come and quietly cover me with a soft blanket. Regardless of the temperature the blanket always seemed to provide just the right coziness to ensure a comfortable nap. Almost without thinking, as a parent, I've done the same for my children.

This afternoon, shortly after lying down on the chesterfield, I felt a blanket being gently tucked around my shoulders. I slowly opened my eyes fully expecting to see Mom. Instead I saw my young son quietly tiptoeing out of the room.

* * *

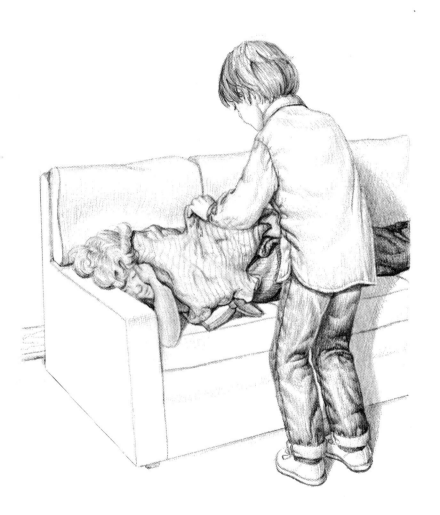

Generosity

Fourteen years of age, watching a curling game in our small town rink, I was approached by a woman, a stranger to me. "You must be Mrs. Lee's daughter," she said. "Well, I just want you to know that your mother is the kindest person I have ever met." I don't know who the woman was or what prompted her remarks. However, I do remember, even at that rebellious age, I heard what she said as a spoken truth.

Despite Mom's growing confusion over the last few years, those traits of generosity and kindness have persisted. Whenever she receives a gift she really likes she will offer it to another family member. It never occurs to her to give away what she doesn't like. Sometimes during the night, she may bring the treasured article into our living space and leave it for us to discover in the morning. Frequently, at mealtimes when she tastes a particular food or beverage she especially enjoys, she will offer it to one of us.

In her gradually narrowing world of perceptions and capabilities, her sensitive awareness of the "other" still remains.

✳   ✳   ✳

Safe-Keeping

Mom has a unique way of taking care of anything she considers especially valuable—she hides it! Under a lace doily, between the leaves of a book, in a china cup, or under the mattress. She hides it, she explains, so she'll know exactly where to find it.

Such safe keeping adds much excitement to her life, engaging her in a perpetual treasure hunt. While the particular sought-after item might not appear for weeks, Mom usually ends each day in triumph. As she cheerfully exclaims, "Isn't it wonderful? I almost always find something I've misplaced while I'm looking for something else!"

✳   ✳   ✳

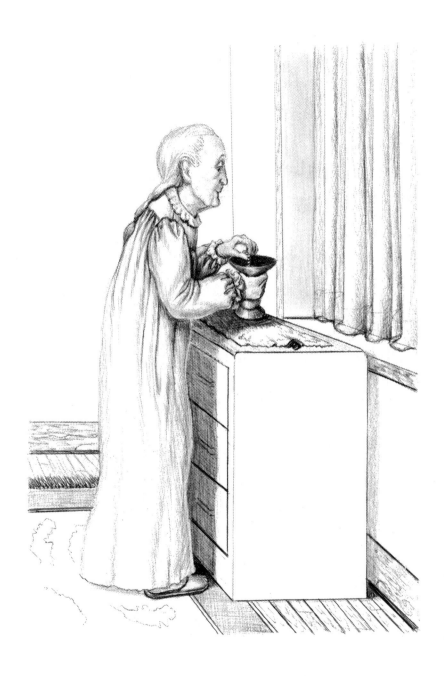

For Both Our Sakes

Must you go out again?"

"Will you be gone long?"

"Two hours! Oh, I'm going to be all alone. Well . . . I guess I'll manage."

"But it's so cold outside. Why don't you just stay home today?"

Steeling myself, I continue my preparations to leave. It's so tempting to remain at home. Yet it is crucial I pursue a life separate from Mom.

I pause, standing at the door. "I promise I'll be home as quickly as I can. Bye, Mom. See you soon."

"Well, yes . . . if I'm still here."

With a pang of guilt, I give her a reassuring hug.

I close the door firmly behind me.

I must go. For both our sakes.

※　　※　　※

In The Now

As long as I can remember, Mom has displayed an appreciation for the "now." It is not uncommon for her, while eating food she likes, to suddenly exclaim, "This is *the best* I've ever tasted!" Or, when looking at something pleasing, to remark, "That's *the prettiest* I've ever seen!"

Her capacity to experience life with freshness was demonstrated in an amusing incident last Sunday. It was one of those rare occasions when all five of our family managed to attend church together. At the conclusion of the service, my husband, who had been sitting four seats away from Mom, waited to escort her back to our car. As Mom approached him, she looked surprised. Smiling warmly, she eagerly grabbed his hand and shaking it said, "Well, hello there. How *wonderful* it is to see you!"

✳   ✳   ✳

The Music Box

Penetrating the animated conversation of my friends, from Mom's room drifts the metallic sound of her music box. "Raindrops Keep Falling On My Head," it cheerfully tinkles. Basking in the warmth of comradeship, I wonder, is the tune calling us for attention or is it simply reflecting one lonely person's way of positively coping with feelings of exclusion?

* * *

D i c k i e

What would you *really* like for your birthday?", I
asked Mom as March 2nd appeared with a flip of the cal-
endar. I waited, half listening, expecting to hear the familiar, "Oh, I don't want a thing, I have everything I
need."

"I'd like a bird. A yellow canary, just like Dickie," Mom
replied with conviction. Dickie had been the little canary
she had tearfully left behind when she emigrated to Canada at the age of twelve. Until now she had never desired
another bird.

And so, on Mom's eighty-fifth birthday "Dickie" moved
in. Dickie with his bright yellow feathers and the promise of being able to sing. And sing he did! His cheery trills
could be heard throughout our home, often accompanied
by the background music of the radio, tuned to the station most pleasing to him. Cage door open, he enjoyed the
expansiveness of Mom's entire room. Flying from place to
place, perching on pictures and plants, he and Mom developed a unique form of communication understood only

by them. When evening came, Mom would beckon him with an outstretched hand on which he'd land and obligingly hop into his cage.

With the opening of Dickie's cage, Mom's door closed. Anyone entering or leaving had to ensure "Boots" was not stalking behind. Boots was our daughter's much loved cat, whose feline whiskers quivered whenever he heard a single chirp.

Despite everyone's watchfulness, on occasion the door was left ajar and Dickie would wing his way out into the entry. This entry opened to the outdoors as well as connecting Mom's room with the rest of the house.

Then, one day it happened. Dickie escaped. Circling in the entry, he was stopped by the swift flick of Boot's claws. Cradled in Mom's hand, he died.

I wondered what Mom would do with all the ambivalent feelings she must have experienced with this untimely death. Not only was she fond of Boots, she absolutely adored her granddaughter. Her resolution was soon revealed in an overheard conversation between she and her friend.

Describing the tragedy, Mom explained, "Dear Boots, he didn't want Dickie to fly outside. He knew he'd perish in the cold. So, he just reached up to try to stop him. But cats have such sharp claws, you know."

Needless to say, Mom, her granddaughter, and 'heroic' Boots were thus able to go on living together with no bad feelings.

* * *

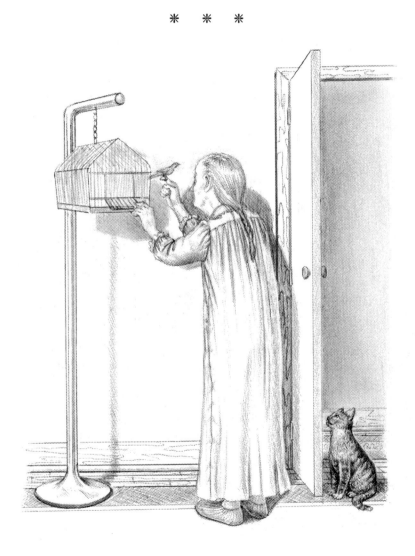

Getting Ready

I discover Mom busily sticking pieces of masking tape on the bottom of her most valued possessions. On the tape she is carefully printing the names of relatives.

Responding to my enquiry she explains, "Well if I should go into a nursing home . . ." I am certain she is not even considering such a move, nor are we. I also know she knows I am not ready to accept the possibility of her death.

Last year when she was quite ill with the flu, I remember one of our friends assuring her how much we all wanted her to recover. Sick as she was, Mom managed to chuckle and replied, "But just think what a terrible world this would be if none of us would leave."

It is true, Mom has always been more accepting of the thought of her death than I have. Only yesterday she chided, "You have to let me go sometime, Judy."

Tears well up in my eyes as I obediently leave her room to find another roll of masking tape.

"Not you, Mom. Not you. Not yet. Please, not yet!"

* * *

S p a c e

I push down hard to tuck in the last freshly laundered nightie. This drawer is crowded. And with good reason! There are only four drawers in this chest and the bottom two are filled with toys—blocks, miniature cars, dolls, puzzles and crayons. They were put there years ago at Mom's invitation. She was delighted when her grandchildren came into her room to play and was pleased when they left some of their favorite toys behind. Frequently they would return to engage her in their pretend games or to cuddle up to her as she read them stories. Loving hours they spent together.

Time has passed. The children have grown into sophisticated teenagers now too big to sit on Nana's lap. Several times I've suggested they move their toys. They're reluctant to do so and can't really say why. I don't demand an explanation sensing a deeper reason for their reluctance than the mere work of such a task.

Mom insists she doesn't need the extra space. "Plenty of room for the toys," she says.

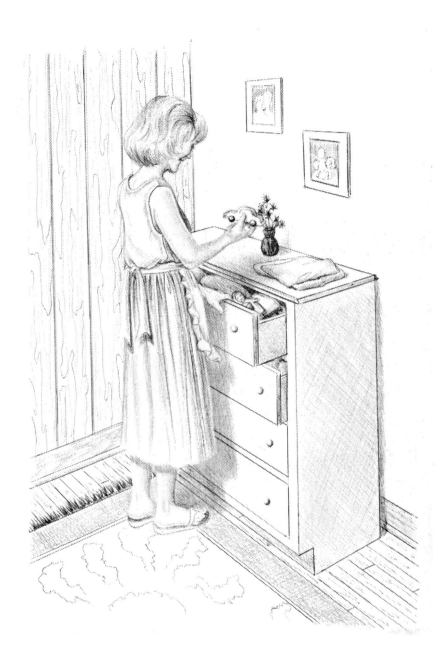

As for me? Well, I'm aware I could take matters into my own hands, clear the drawers and pack away the toys. It certainly would make things more convenient. Yet I know I won't. After all, as a Chinese proverb might express it, "Much room in heart does not necessarily space in drawers make!"

*　*　*

Red Geraniums

Only this morning, when I left to go shopping, I noticed the geranium at the front of the house was finally blooming. A large, bright, scarlet blossom—satisfying sight to a novice gardener like myself.

Now, tasks accomplished, returning home, I glance expectantly at the flower bed, anticipating another wave of pleasure. I gasp and stare in disbelief. The flower is gone! I feel angry, oh so angry! Why can't I grow flowers like my neighbors? It's not fair!

I suspect the geranium's fate.

Better not go in the house just yet.

I begin walking briskly down the street. One, two, three blocks. By the fourth block my anger is beginning to dissipate. My steps become softer, slower. I recall sun-filled days on the farm decades ago. Mom would leave her chores to take me wild flower picking. Buttercups, marsh-marigolds, Indian-paint-brushes, brown-eyed susans, lady slippers—our favorites. As the bitter prairie snowstorms railed, closing all roads to town, it was the bright geranium standing bravely in the bay window that added cheer to all those dark and sometimes lonely winter days.

"Geraniums are such hardy plants; don't freeze easily even with the draft. The pink are pretty but red are sure my favorite," Mom would remark as she shoved more wood into the kitchen stove. Playing with my dolls beside the warm chimney, I'd listen quietly to her comments.

"Strange how so much of life changes yet how some things stay the same," I muse as I near the house.

I am aware my inner turmoil has subsided.

I go inside.

As always Mom is there to greet me.

Wordlessly, I reach out and secure the bright red blossom dangling precariously from her buttonhole.

We look at each other and smile.

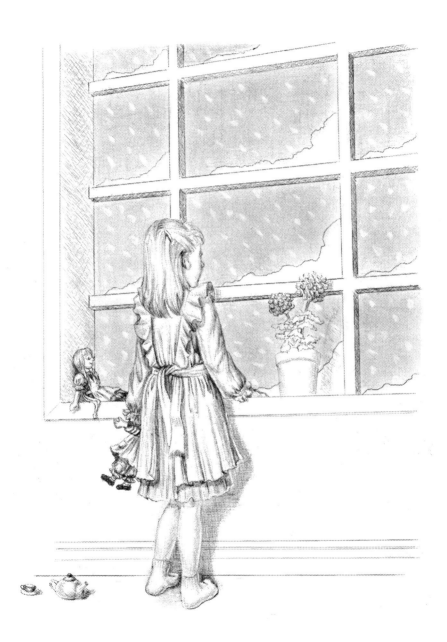

J o g g e r s

Driving together in the car, we pass a woman jogging.

"She must be in a hurry to get some place," Mom comments dryly.

I smile, realizing for the first time how Mom must have been viewing the numerous joggers we have encountered daily in our travels. With the modern emphasis on physical fitness, much of the population must appear to her to be constantly rushing, with a definite, urgent destination in mind!

❋　❋　❋

An Adventure

Mom! Mom! Mom!"

Where is she? I can't find her! I rush to the stairway and look with dread down to the bottom. Thank God, she's not there! A frantic search from room to room reveals no trace of her. Other family members are alerted. We begin to search the streets. Concerned neighbors join us.

Where could she have gone? She used to boast that despite her other limitations she was still pretty good on her "pins" as she referred to her short sturdy legs. But still, how could she possibly travel so fast? Unless . . . Oh, no! I mustn't think such things. I run home and phone the local police station.

"Just a moment, please. Yes . . . someone did call in about an elderly lady. She was wandering along the street. Heavy traffic there. They were afraid she might get hit by a car. She didn't seem to know where she lived so the constable took her downtown to the Social Services Office."

"Oh, no, I'll bet some of my former students work here," my husband mutters as we approach the building.

We find Mom quite intact. Only her crimson hat is a bit askew. She looks pleased to see us. She needs no coaxing to hurry off to the closest washroom with me. The staff are friendly. Sure enough, some do know my husband. They're surprised and amused to make the connection. They affectionately say their good-byes to Mom.

Just as we're about to go out the door, one calls, "Thanks for singing to us, Mrs. Lee." Mom nods, smiles and waves. My husband and I look at each other. We both know Mom has quite a repertoire of songs. We don't stop to ask any further questions.

Seated between us in the car Mom exudes a new sparkle. She's become more articulate, responding to our comments with words she hasn't remembered for months.

In celebration of her safe return we all go out to eat. Despite our weariness, it's impossible not to be cheered by Mom's exhilaration. No doubt about it, she's enjoyed her experience immensely.

✳   ✳   ✳

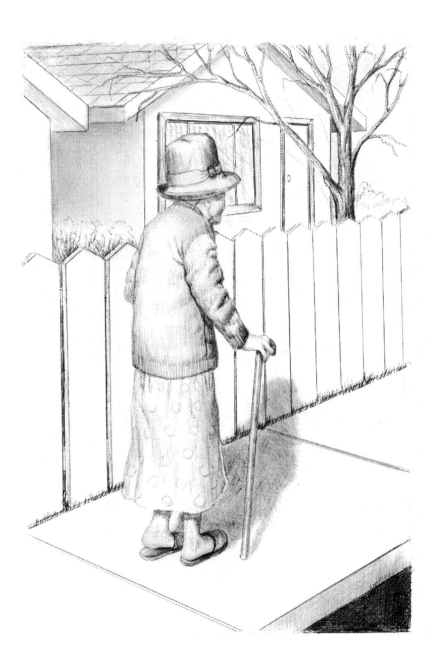

Care-Giving

O h, thank you! You're so good to me." Mom looks grateful as I put her slippers on and bring her a cup of hot coffee in her favorite cup.

I know she appreciates what I do. I also doubt she has any memory of what I did for her yesterday. Tomorrow she will have little recollection of what transpired between us today. We live strictly in the "now."

Mom has also lost much of her ability to communicate. It is unlikely she will even be able to tell anyone else whether I am gentle or rough with her. She is completely entrusted to my care. Sometimes this responsibility weighs heavily. I feel both powerful and helpless.

I must remind myself I do have the freedom of choice. Do I become a martyr who does what she has to do with resentment? Or, do I view these tasks as privileges and respond with humility and love?

Within the confines of this home, and in the everydayness of my life are challenging opportunities for personal growth. This situation demands I re-examine all my motives for caregiving. It necessitates an honest answer to the question, "Who am I really, when nobody is looking?"

Commitment

We are all dressed up and ready to go. Looking forward to the party—close friends, colleagues, interesting people. It promises to be a most pleasurable evening.

My husband proceeds out to the car while I go to check on Mom one last time before leaving.

Uneasiness creeps over me when I see her. Although not complaining, she does not look very well. Her breathing seems somewhat labored. Immediately I feel disappointed and conflicted.

My husband is already in the driver's seat patiently waiting. He has grown accustomed to my last minute checking. With a heavy heart I explain why I feel I simply cannot attend the party. He offers to stay home too but I decline, urging him to go and enjoy himself.

As the car pulls out of the driveway, I experience a great sense of relief. I go back into the house to reassure Mom, I will be home for the evening.

I am confident, once at the party, my husband will enjoy himself. I am also confident although he may prefer my company, he will bear me no resentment. Nor, upon his return, will he shower me with unwanted pity. He knows me well. He understands that tonight I have chosen to be where I most need and want to be.

Thank God for the nature of our marriage.

Two Teachers

How are you today Mrs. Lee?"

"Oh, I'm fine except I'm getting old."

"Well, that's good because we know what the other alternative is, don't we?"

They both laugh. It's their own private joke they've shared on previous occasions.

I look with gratitude at our friend. Just as she once embraced my children when they were small, in more recent years, she's extended her interest and care to Mom.

Mom eagerly returns the affection. Every lunchtime she carefully stores the wrapped soda crackers she gets from Meals On Wheels in a special jar. "For Kay's children," she reminds me. "They get hungry in school. It's a long day for little ones."

It's been many years since Mom taught school but she's able to listen appreciatively as Kay recounts amusing classroom incidents. Then, haltingly from the recesses of her mind emerge her own memories. One room country schoolhouses with pot bellied stoves; inspectors who came unannounced; blizzards that blew snow drifts up to the window sills; Christmas concerts in which everyone participated; appreciative parents and best of all, beloved pupils.

Kay, patiently and attentively listens to Mom's recollections. It is obvious decades separate them only in age. They still are able to communicate. Teacher to teacher. Heart to heart.

* * *

Priorities

Phone calls to make; clothes to be washed; business to attend to; a meal to prepare—the day just doesn't seem long enough! And there is Mom alone in her room. Except for taking care of necessities, I've hardly talked to her today. Her loneliness seems to seep from under her door and stalk me in my busyness. "Tough jelly beans" as my children would say, I simply don't have time to give her any special attention right now. This report must be written and mailed. Besides, I want to accomplish at least one thing of lasting value before the day is over.

Exasperated at not finding the necessary information to write the report, as a last resort I rush to the filing cabinet. Perhaps in one of my more organized moments I actually put what I'm looking for right where it belongs.

Impatiently flipping through the files, one labelled IMPORTANT PAPERS catches my attention. Curiously I pull it out. Inside is a document pertaining to bequeathing one's body to the Division of Morphological Science. Dated 1977, it bears Mom's signature.

Yes, I remember the time well. It was the year of my husband's sabbatical when he planned to do research in Europe. The children and I were excited at the prospect of accompanying him. Mom was not in the best of health. Her concern, however, was not that we would be leaving her behind but that our much-looked-forward-to-trip might be curtailed should she die when we were overseas. Despite our protests, she obtained the documents from the medical school and convinced my husband to co-sign them.

I recall her saying, "There, dear, I'm glad that's done. Now if something should happen to me while you're away, I don't want you to spoil your trip by coming home early. I've been told the university will arrange a nice little memorial service later at your convenience."

Thoughtfully I replace the file and push the cabinet drawer shut. The report can wait. It's lost its priority.

Mom's face brightens as I enter her room carrying two cups of freshly brewed coffee.

Curled up in a chair across from her, I study her kindly face. I sense myself in the presence of a wise teacher. I take a deep relaxing breath. I know I still have much to learn.

* * *

Keeping Current

From the time I can remember, Mom has always possessed an eagerness for learning and a willingness to change. I can still picture her sitting in the middle of our farm kitchen, while white long underwear steamed in the boiler on the wood stove, pausing to read with interest some article in the latest Farmer's Free Press Weekly.

After my Dad died and Mom was left alone to fix whatever broke around the house, I recall her being very satisfied with her accomplishments. "You learn something new every day," she frequently remarked.

This openness to change continued into later years. She was well into her eighties when, one day, waiting for her to sign her pension cheque, I glanced over her shoulder. At first I thought she had just forgotten how to write "Mrs." Then, to my delight, I realized she had not meant to write "Mrs." at all. Indeed, as a woman of the Age of Aquarius, she had purposely written "Ms."!

* * *

Separate Lives

She sits waiting, ready, all dressed up in one of her favorite outfits. She still likes to wear a hat even though all her hats have become too large. From underneath the brim her soulful eyes peer out, her gaze following me as I move about the room.

"You could come with me. Why don't you come? Sure, you come!"

Mom's voice is coaxing.

The taxi will soon arrive to take her to the local senior citizen's centre. There's a weekly afternoon program designed for shut-ins. A valuable, much needed service.

"No, Mom, I don't think so. This is your group, and I don't want to intrude. You go by yourself and have a good time."

She looks disappointed.

I know she wants me to accompany her. But I am reluctant. I need some time alone. Besides, I don't want her treated as a bystander. And that's what seems to happen when we go out together in public. Other people tend to talk to me and ignore her. Despite my good intentions, I

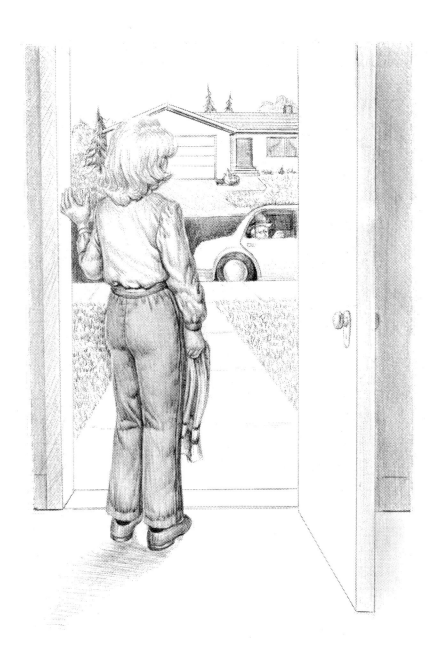

end up speaking for both of us. Well, I am determined that won't happen this time. This must remain her exclusive group.

I stand at the window and wave as the taxi pulls away. She is unable to see me. But I see her. Lone little figure sitting in the back seat barely tall enough to look out.

A lump comes to my throat.

I turn away from the window, unsure I've made the right decision.

The house feels empty.

* * *

W e a l t h

We had just returned from an evening service in the chapel when Mom told me she had a confession to make. I was about eleven years old at the time.

"Tonight, right before the collection plate was passed I looked into my purse. I found only a penny. I realized it was all I had left after paying the month's bills. One little penny. I remembered the story in the Bible of the widow's mite . . . how she gave what she had and was blessed. Yet, even with the knowledge of that parable, I simply could not get myself to put my one penny into the empty collection plate. Perhaps I would have been braver if I hadn't been the first in the row. Anyway, I was too proud. I hope God forgives me."

I don't recall my response. I doubt if I said anything. To me my mother was Goodness personified and I was certain God, too, regarded her as such—penny or no penny.

Before, and since that time, Mom has worked hard, often without monetary compensation; always without complaint. In recent years her meagre government pension has provided the most financial security she has ever known.

Today, having cashed her cheque, I return home and count out her money for her. As I turn to leave, she calls me back. In her outstretched hand is a crisp twenty dollar bill.

"For you. Buy yourself a treat on me."

Her eyes sparkle. She exudes a sense of wealth greater than any millionaire I've ever met.

Our familiar game begins. She counters each of my refusals with a convincing argument about how well-off she really is. Eventually, our game concludes when I gratefully accept her gift.

As I turn to go, she is busily searching for a safe place to stow her cash. I smile to myself, filled with the sensation I am, in fact, leaving the presence of one of the world's richest women.

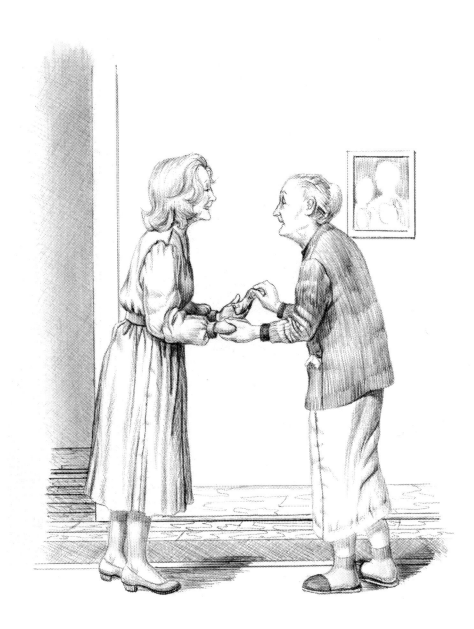

Her Place

Mom is sound asleep. Sitting here at her bedside, I look around her colorful room filled with keepsakes.

A small grey granite coffee pot brought from her childhood home on the Minnesota prairies.

Numerous snapshots of friends, children, grandchildren and great grandchildren.

A green cut-glass candy dish once belonging to my sister. She had bought it with the twenty-five cents earned from selling a syrup pail of wild strawberries to travellers on the highway.

Plants.

An electric stove and fridge, both disconnected now. The elements of the stove covered with residue of melted utensils.

A wall plaque with raised letters, "In what time I am afraid I will trust, Psalm 56:3." Often during my growing up years, at times of crisis, I recall Mom fortifying herself by reading aloud that verse.

Ornaments ordered by me, $1.09 C.O.D. from the Eaton's Christmas catalogue. I was nine years old then—the year "we" taught school together in northern Manitoba.

A dresser.

Mom's family portrait taken when she was only five—eleven girls and two boys. All gone now, Mom the sole survivor.

A tattered piece of paper with a poem dated 1943 scrawled by my brother from the front lines in Germany.

Many, many books.

A sewing machine once used to mend all our clothes.

Greeting cards: Christmas, Mother's Day, birthday, Valentine's—the season is unimportant. Whenever I've attempted to take the old ones down, Mom has convinced me it is their brightness and message that really matter.

A radio.

Our old cat dozing on the bed confident his comfort will be respected. Beside him lies a large doll looking equally comfortable. I remember when my daughter was small, after having observed her Nana relating to her dolls, came to whisper in my ear, "Nana thinks they're real." I could understand why she would get that impression, yet I have always known even as Mom covers and uncovers the dolls and props them up to sit for the day,

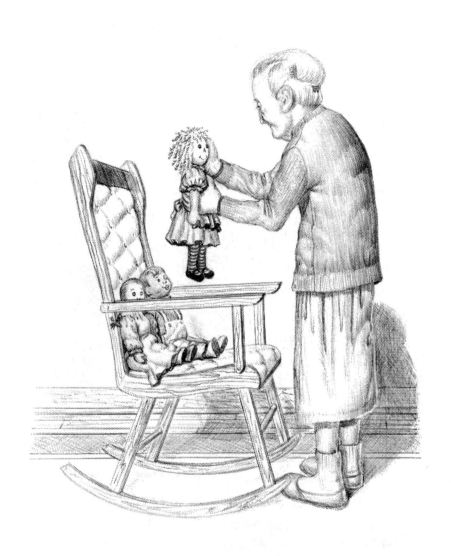

she realizes they are only toys. At the same time they provide an opportunity for her to continue to express her nurturing, child-loving self.

A black and white T.V.

A well-worn Bible on her bedside table. No longer able to read it herself, it is as though its very presence provides a source of wisdom, comfort and promise of eternity. Opening it now I discover Mom has written in the fly-leaf.

April 1st '79

My sister Edith has passed away. I'll always remember how, when I wept in the alley—the yellow flowers given me. Our gate opened for me. Kindness shown me by my friends. Thank You All.

* * *

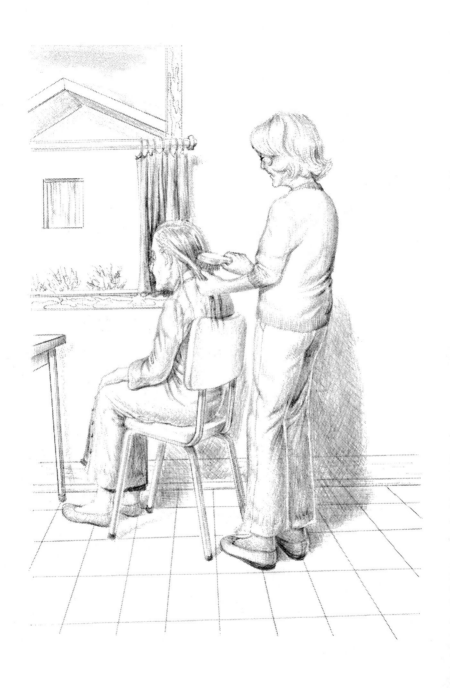

T u r n i n g   P o i n t

O ver the decades, Mom's two thick, black braids
have gradually diminished to one thinner, white braid.
Until recently, each morning she has been in the habit of
combing and braiding her hair, then carefully pinning it
up and securing it with a hairnet.

As I now look at her dishevelled appearance, I am
forced to acknowledge we have reached another turning
point. Although she still manages to dress herself, this is
the second consecutive day she's neglected to comb her
hair. It's true, I am reluctant to assume yet another daily
task, even more painful for me to accept, however, is
Mom's decreasing ability to take care of herself.

Her hair is tangled and without thinking I begin
brushing too briskly. She winces.

Brush suspended, my mind flashes back to my childhood when my long, fine, blond hair was braided into two
pigtails tied with bright ribbons. How I loved the ribbons
and hated the combing! What might have been even
more of a dreaded ordeal became tolerable only because,

as Mom coaxed out the snarls with water, she told me a continued story. We made it up together as we went along.

The memory fades and I begin to brush Mom's hair again—this time more slowly, more gently. I can sense her relaxing.

"Mom, remember when I was little and you . . . "

We both chuckle.

Tomorrow I'll buy some bright pink combs. They'll show up nicely. And, yes, a new hairnet. This one has a hole in it.

＊　＊　＊

Well - Meaning

While attending a community function, an acquaintance comes over to say hello. She's an energetic, caring woman and I am pleased to see her. Her greeting is familiar; one I've heard from others.

"I had hoped to come and visit your mother this week but the time just went. Of course, I know she is well taken care of by you and your family. She's so lucky to have you."

She looks genuinely apologetic and I believe what she says. No doubt she means well. Naturally she is preoccupied with her own life and meeting more obvious needs. I really do understand, so outwardly I accept her explanation without protest. Yet inwardly I am helplessly screaming, "We need you. We are family; we can never represent the outside world to Mom. You do. She needs to know she's not forgotten, that she is still important to people like yourself. Family can never take your place."

*   *   *

A Guest

She's the first to arrive. She's been here many times before. Knows us well enough to dress comfortably when she comes. After all, she expects our dogs to greet her enthusiastically. But this time it's obvious she's taken special care in her dress. She's dressed brightly and expensively, right from her fourteen-karat gold earrings down to her Italian made shoes. She looks absolutely elegant.

Mom notices immediately. "My that's pretty . . . what you've got on!"

Our friend laughs appreciatively. I realize she has anticipated Mom's response. Over the years she's become aware of how much Mom likes color and pretty clothes. Of course, she knows, even today she would have been most welcome in her "grubbies" but despite her busy schedule, she's put a lot of thought and time into her ensemble.

I am grateful for her effort. It is one of her unique, endearing ways of adding to this very important 90th Birthday celebration.

✳   ✳   ✳

Family Bonds

The phone rings. It's Sunday. I glance at the clock. Yes, I think I know who is calling.

"Hello," I answer expectantly.

Seconds tick by. Then haltingly comes the sound of my oldest brother's voice. Incapacitated by multiple sclerosis, he now is completely bedridden, unable to even hold the phone himself. His weakened lungs make his breathing more labored, his speaking difficult. Fortunately he has a devoted wife and family to care for him and assist him in making these weekly long distance calls.

Painstakingly, yet with flashes of humor, he enquirers about each member of the family by name.

"I'm fine," he says in response to my expression of concern. I, who will complain aloud about even a slight headache, decide not to voice my disbelief.

Then comes his familiar question—the primary reason for his call.

"How is Mom? Is Mom there?"

"She's doing really well. Sitting here with us in the living room. I'll let you talk to her."

"It's your son, Doug," I explain as she stiffly and slowly makes her way to the phone. "Use your strong voice now."

Mom accepts the receiver, unsure which end to speak into.

"Hello" she murmurs.

"Louder, Mom. Otherwise Doug can't hear you."

"Hello" she obligingly repeats with more volume.

Except for the occasional "yah," she says little else. It's obvious, however, from her expression she knows she's speaking to her first-born, the son who arrived on Mother's Day over fifty years ago. As she listens her face seems to soften and her eyes brighten.

Observing her I am again reminded how bonds of love endure, surpass all physical limitations and by only a few words span time and distance.

❋   ❋   ❋

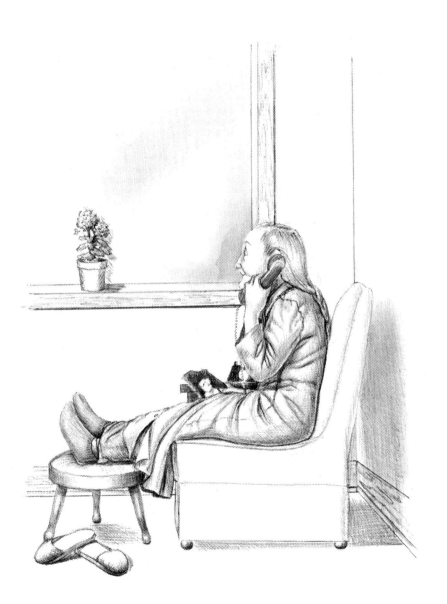

L o s s

Life is harsh at times. Today I felt criticized and rejected.

The house is quiet when I arrive home. Only Mom here. She must be in her room. Like a vulnerable youngster with hurt feelings, I find myself seeking her out.

There she is, seated on her rumpled bed. Her unaware gaze warns me not to risk disclosing my pain. Looking at her, I once more feel like an abandoned child. Longing for the comforting mother of earlier years, I sit down and put my arm around her. She remains unresponsive, not noticing my tears. My only solace comes from trusting that locked within her frail body still lives the person who has always loved me. Who, I know, if able to express herself, would reassure me all will be well.

I reach in and take a hankie from her housecoat pocket. For some unknown reason, I am reluctant to leave her side.

The afternoon sunlight gradually fades. The rest of the family will soon be home. I must go and make supper.

❋   ❋   ❋

Recorded Memories

Born in a log house on the Minnesota prairie; emigrating to Canada at the turn of the century; she became a pioneer teacher, wife and mother. A gifted story teller, Mom could enrapture any audience as she recounted her experiences.

Fortunately; when she was sixty-five we decided to record on tape four hours of her recollections as well as some of the songs she used to sing to amuse her children. At the time it seemed an enjoyable yet relatively unimportant task for the feeling was that Mom and her stories would always be available to us. Such was not the case. As Mom aged, her stories became more infrequent and eventually ceased altogether.

Twenty years later the tapes were recovered from a dusty box stored in the back of a closet. What a joy to observe Mom as she listened to them for the very first time! Her vacant expression slowly changed to a soft smile of recognition. Every once in awhile she would nod her head affirmatively. Occasionally she would sing along or finish telling us the story.

Since then, the tapes have been played many times. More valuable than any "talking" library book, they have enabled Mom to overcome the barrier imposed by hardening arteries and to reconnect with her "meaning full" past. Originally intended as a gift to her children and grandchildren, her recorded songs and stories have now become a gift to herself.

✳　　✳　　✳

A Long Trip

Sceptics might say we should not have come . . . long, expensive and tiring air travel, for one reason. And ever since we arrived Mom 's been acting as if Milton, her youngest son, is just sleeping in that coffin. Her daughter-in-law has been most understanding—bless her kind heart. Not only that, prior to the service, Mom and I spent most of the time holed up in the funeral-parlour's bathroom, washing her lingerie. An "accident" on the way. Thank goodness for sufficient time and warm running water. My own fault—I should have taken precautions in dressing her. But I detest putting those bulky things on Mom.

Well, that's all behind us now and we are back at my sister-in-law's home sharing memories of my brother. I'm sorry Mom can't join in our recollection. If she could I'm sure she'd be telling us about the time when Milton was a toddler, fell into the rain barrel, almost drowned, and when they dried him with towels warmed in the oven, they discovered he had curly hair. Or the time he got a twenty-two shell caught in his windpipe. Or the time . . .

Marvellous stories—repeated often—etched in our memories! He certainly was a loved and important member of our family.

Was I wrong to bring her here? No one seems offended by her lack of awareness. I'm very grateful for their acceptance. I watch her now across the living room, sitting there looking cosy and content. Grandchildren on either side with arms around her, her aged face framed between two younger, saddened faces. Ever since we arrived there have been many loving arms to hug her, hold her and patiently guide her. They've been reminding her of times years ago when she let them bake cookies or when she brought them hot cocoa in bed.

Yes, all in all, I'm thankful we've made this trip. Even though this is a sad occasion there is also cause for celebration. A celebration of how love continues to be passed from one generation to another to another and back again.

✳   ✳   ✳

S t a f f o r d

We found Stafford car-hopping at the drive-in restaurant in Winnipeg. Or rather, Stafford found us.

From the vantage point of our car we had watched this unusual, big tomcat jump on the hood of several other cars and peer through their windshields. Eventually he came to our car, jumped up; looked in at us; then surprised us by walking around to our open window, hopping in onto my husbands knee, lying down and falling quickly asleep. Of course we took him home with us. Enquiries and newspaper ads failed to locate his original owner.

Stafford exuded dignity. His very presence commanded respect. After Mom came to live with us, she and Stafford developed a special bond. In fact Stafford literally moved in with Mom. He slept comfortably on her bed which, if he preferred to snooze in the morning, remained unmade so as not to disturb him. It was not unusual for Mom to serve him warmed milk in a china saucer wherever he was sitting.

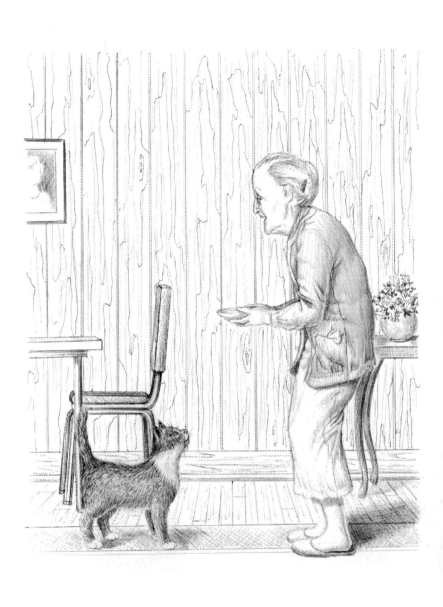

As Stafford grew older, lost his teeth, shed more fur and developed halitosis the rest of us avoided most physical contact with him. Not Mom. Stafford continued to seek her out, confident he would always be welcome on her knee and lovingly petted.

One week it became evident Stafford's health was declining. Since he didn't seem to be suffering we decided not to take him to the vet. Instead, we all did what we could to make him comfortable.

It seemed very fitting that in Mom's room, stretched out on the rug in front of the heater with a china saucer of milk beside him, he died. He was twenty-two years old.

With the exception of Mom, we all cried.

✳   ✳   ✳

Our Friend

How will it be, if I come over on my lunch hour once a week and visit with your Mom? I really am fond of her, you know. Besides, I've always wished I could have spent more time with my own dear Nannie, and your Mom, in certain ways, reminds me of her."

My friend sounds sincere in her offer. She's heard me fret over how inadequate I sometimes feel to dispel Mom's apparent loneliness. While recognizing she may be inconveniencing herself, I now gratefully accept her offer.

And so she comes. Week after week. Faithfully.

Mom begins to look forward to her arrival. Getting dressed now assumes more of a purpose.

In preparation, I set the small table in Mom's room, making sure to include the pepper and salt. After all, although Meals on Wheels are nutritious, they're not known for their spiciness.

I interrupt their lunch only to bring in hot coffee. My friend and I speak little to each other. We both acknowledge, without saying, that this is definitely Mom's time.

As I go about my daily tasks, I can hear murmurs of their conversation. I feel lighter. My friend. Our friend. Indeed, the blessing of her presence permeates our entire home. It drifts out from Mom's room to comfort me like a warm shawl around my shoulders.

✳　✳　✳

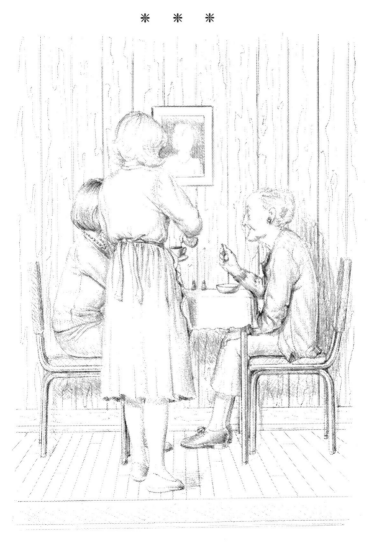

N e e d e d

She sits there in her housecoat. Hands folded idly in her lap. No longer able to walk briskly, wash clothes, mend, cook, or lend a helping hand wherever needed. No longer even able to speak words of wisdom or encouragement.

She sits there staring sadly into space. This daughter, this wife, this mother, this grandmother, this great grandmother who has made her whole purpose in life to serve others, now feels useless. Willing spirit trapped in an aged body.

How can I let her know that despite her limitations, she is still wanted, still needed?

I curl up beside her on the chesterfield. "Mom, my feet are cold. Would you mind if I stretched out and put them in your lap?"

Wordlessly, she lifts the blanket covering her knees. As I tuck my feet underneath, her lotion-smooth hands gently yet firmly grasp my toes. A soft smile of contentment creeps across her dear wrinkled face. She looks knowingly at me. Still wanted, still needed, still useful.

※　　※　　※

The Apron

From time to time, Mom develops a special attachment to a particular article of clothing. Most recently it has been a bright, multi-colored, flowered apron with red lace trim. She likes to wear it morning, noon and sometimes even to bed.

Today, prior to taking her out to a restaurant, I suggested she take her apron off for the occasion. She complied, giving no outward objection. We left home looking prim and proper.

Now later this evening, I am assisting her in getting ready to retire. Off comes her sweater, her dress, her petticoat, and there in all it's bright glory, is her apron neatly tied!

✳   ✳   ✳

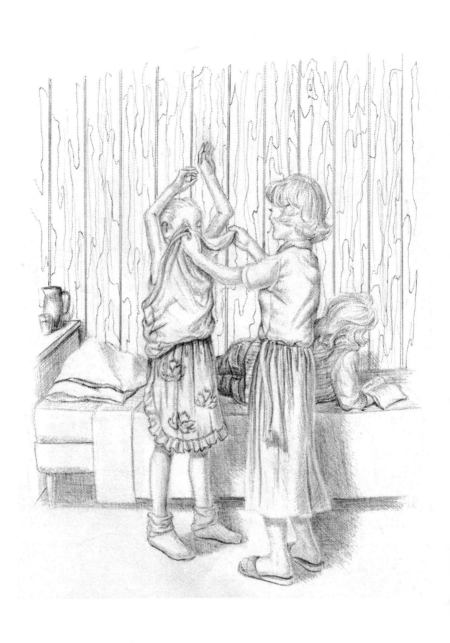

Forgiveness

She walked the floors with him as a newborn baby.

She patiently held the towels while I, an un-experienced mother, struggled to bathe him.

She rocked him, sang to him, read to him, talked to him and loved him. Oh, how she loved this grandson of hers! And he loved her back.

Many years they delighted in each other's company. But, gradually, as she became more confused and he became more factual, their relationship deteriorated.

"No, Nana, you're wrong! That's not true!," he'd yell, his ten-year-old face flushed with exasperation.

"Yes it is! I know what I'm talking about!," she'd retort, desperate to hide her declining clarity of mind.

I felt powerless to change the situation. My heart ached whenever I heard the slamming doors and raised voices.

With growing maturity he confronted less and became patronizingly tolerant of her confusion. She avoided him whenever possible.

Then, at sixteen, he decided he was ready and it was time to be nice to his Nana again. He began giving her kind attention, hugging her, and going into her room to wish her good-night before she fell asleep.

With no sign of bitterness, she responded warmly to his overtures, frequently following him around the house.

One evening my husband and I returned home at midnight to find our son seated on the couch watching a home video with one arm around his girlfriend and the other around his Nana. Mom barely glanced at us as we came in, no doubt fearful we might interrupt her obvious enjoyment.

During the past months I have marvelled at her seeming ability to forgive her grandson for all his rude behavior of the past. Cynically, I have wondered if she was able to be far more forgiving than I could ever be, simply because she just couldn't remember the hurts. Today I learned otherwise.

They were sitting together watching a television program of particular interest to him. Mom starts to babble incoherently—a behavior she's begun to use when she wants attention and can't find the words to express herself.

"Nana, be quiet, I can't hear!" He speaks more firmly and louder than usual.

Her eyes open wide with surprise. She stops her senseless chatter, puts her gnarled hand on his arm and leans forward turning her head so she can see his face.

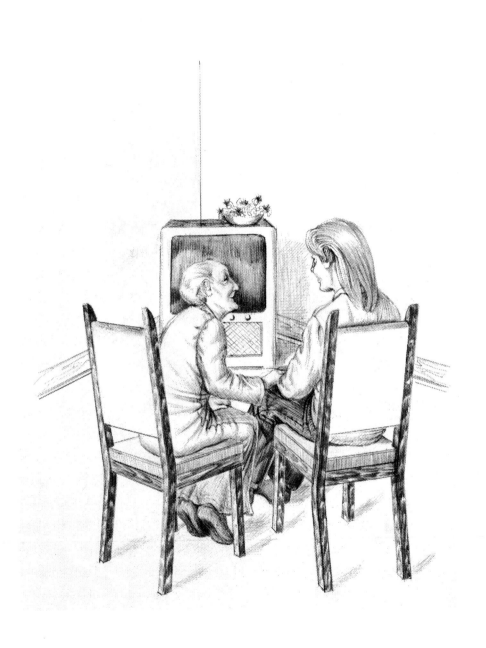

"No, but I thought you were being so good to me!" Her voice is strong. She speaks clearly, convincingly.

The T.V. momentarily forgotten, he looks at her, says nothing, then smiles. His young shoulders shift slightly as though freed from a heavy burden. They sit there in silence.

Side by side. Elder and youth. Forgiving and forgiven.

The Right To Know

It was only a couple of weeks ago when he phoned. He was coming West in the spring. "Looking forward to the trip", he said. We'd have some fun times, my brother and I. Then the unexpected long distance call came, shattering our plans. He had been discovered dead in his apartment—cause of death unknown.

Engulfed in my grief, I look across the room at Mom. During the past months, she has said little, speaking only in monosyllables and seeming oblivious to most of the world around her. She sits there now, quietly, almost peacefully. Unaware of her son's death; insulated from the loss. She's known so much pain, why should she suffer more? If I don't tell her no one else will. I hate possessing such power of censorship!

Her unawareness gives me time. Time to cry. Time to think. Time to realize Mom has a right to know. Even if she might not comprehend the message, I must tell her.

I kneel on the floor so she can see me. I take her hands in mine. She looks at me vacantly. I speak slowly.

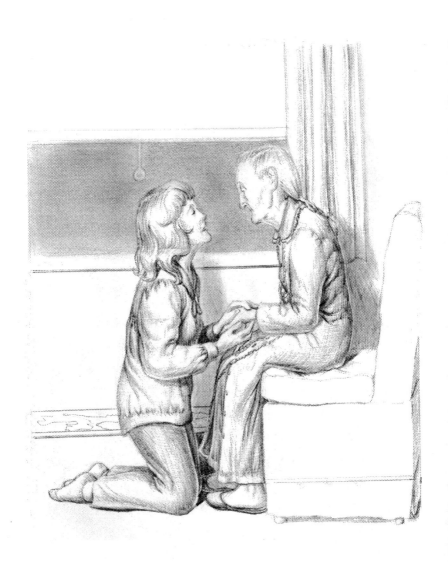

"Mom, I have something to tell you. Your son, Raymond . . . you remember Raymond, he was the one who . . ." I continue, hoping something might register in her mind. "Mom, Raymond has died. I'm sorry. I know you love him and I know he loved you very much."

I wait. She remains still and mute. I wonder if she's understood me. I watch her face for some sign of recognition. Nothing. Then, ever so slowly, two big tears appear and roll down her wrinkled cheeks. I climb up on the couch and put my arms around her frail little shoulders. We sit there alone—close together.

✳   ✳   ✳

An Accident

I was right there when it happened. Right next to Mom on the stairway. She turned. I knew she was falling and I couldn't catch her. I felt so helpless.

Now she's in pain. No visible broken bones. A cracked rib perhaps? It's the weekend and the doctor's office is closed. Out-patient emergency usually means a long wait. Would it be worth the effort and the suffering? I long for the old days when the doctor made home visits.

I decide to settle for telephone consultation and suggested pills to ease her discomfort. Tomorrow we'll slowly go through all the necessary procedures—driving, getting in and out of the car, undressing, examination, x-rays. We'll do them, unsure of the benefits, but not wanting to omit anything that might be helpful. I dread it.

But today. What about today? She is obviously hurting. Not much I can do . . . yes, there is one thing I can do. Past experience has taught me being in pain is an isolating, lonely experience.

Sitting here close beside her I feel somewhat better. I trust in even a small way she does too.

✳   ✳   ✳

C h a n g e s

This morning I spread the jelly on the toast before giving it to Mom.

Last month I put the jelly on her plate and the knife in her hand.

Two months ago I only put the jelly on her plate.

Before Christmas I called her attention to the spoon in the jelly jar.

Last year I simply set the table and left it up to her.

Before that she made her own breakfast.

Today I spread the jelly on her toast.

*　　*　　*

A Necessary Break

Y ou are going on another holiday? And leaving Mom? . . . . Well, yes, I'm sure you think this woman you've hired will take good care of her. But she's not family, you know. Mom's going to miss you."

I can hear the edge in my brother's voice. Of course, I can understand he's concerned. No doubt he feels powerless to remedy the situation from such a distance.

I don't even attempt to articulate my feelings. I am very weary. How can I explain to him that it's not really Mom I want to leave? I simply know I need a break. A break from the anxiety I experience every time I leave the house; the readiness to cope with any emergency; the listening in the night. However, most of all, as I observe Mom becoming more frail, I am desperate to escape the constant, painful reminder I am losing her.

With a heavy heart, I hang up the receiver and continue to pack.

* * *

L e a v i n g

Finally the car is packed. We are all set to go. Just as we are backing out of the driveway I feel a desperate urge to see Mom one more time.

"Wait! I just need to run back into the house for a minute."

My husband patiently puts the car in Park. I can hear our son and daughter sigh in exasperation. No one says anything.

She is where I left her; her stooped frail figure sitting on the bed.

How I long for the old days when, by now, she would have been waving at the window, smiling, letting me know in every possible way she was happy I was taking a vacation.

Repeating my good-bye, I search her face, hoping for some indication she is accepting of my leaving. Instead, her eyes remain unfocused. She seems in a world all her own. Is she hurt? Is she angry? I have no idea. Deep down inside, I wonder if I will ever see her here again. I must not entertain such fears! I must leave, the family is waiting. I give her one last kiss.

As we drive away I feel like a mother abandoning her small child to the care of a stranger.

This prospective holiday certainly seems bittersweet.

* * *

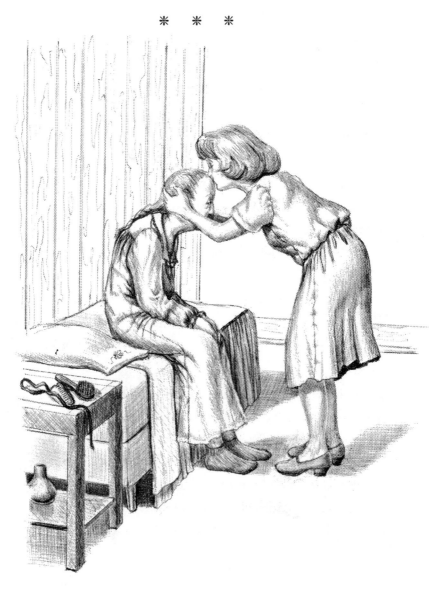

Circle of Friends

Icould have phoned earlier but I didn't. In fact, I could
have phoned daily but I didn't. Now as I push the dial
buttons my hand trembles. I can feel my heart pound as I
wait for my friend to answer.

"Your care person called me and I went over. We decided to hospitalize your Mom. I hope that is all right
with you. She had stopped eating and drinking and consequently was dehydrated. Your doctor actually came to
your house to see her. He recommended she be put on in-
travenous."

I feel cold with fear. I mumble something about my
brother and family expecting we will visit them on our
way home. We will now need to decide whether or not to
change our plans.

If shocked at my response, our friend hides it well.
"Okay Judy, you think about it and phone me back. I've
contacted a number of your other friends and we're taking turns sitting with your mother at the hospital. You
don't have to worry that she will be left alone."

Of course given time to overcome the shock and with
my brother's encouragement we decide to return home

immediately. After a phone consultation with Mom's doctor, I choose to continue to travel by car with my family rather than fly alone. I sense I need time to prepare for what I anticipate may be ahead.

Silently speeding across the miles, in the midst of my tears, I am deeply comforted by the close presence of my family and the image of Mom watched over by loving friends.

On Guard

I remember now . . . it was when they made their morning rounds. The younger nurse had looked questioningly when her superior suggested a particular medical procedure—as though she wanted to protest but didn't dare. Shortly afterwards they returned and ushered me out of the room.

Standing in the hallway, I listened helplessly to Mom's protest. When I am allowed to re-enter her room, I find Mom still distressed. Obviously something has been done to her she has not liked.

Why did I not question what they were planning to do? Why did I once again give away my powers to medical authority? Now I can only apologize to Mom and promise her I will not let it happen again.

A laboratory technician enters. He explains he has an order to take another blood sample. I tell him, "No."

Looking relieved, almost grateful, he obediently turns and leaves. I can hear the empty tubes rattle in his case as he proceeds down the hospital corridor.

✳   ✳   ✳

Night Vigil

How I hate going to sleep at times of great distress! I yearn to stay vigilantly alert for I dread those first moments upon awakening. Those moments when I am flooded with the realization of the actual situation. This morning is no exception. My first thought of making Mom breakfast is immediately overcome with the awareness her room is empty, she's no longer here, she's lying helplessly alone in a hospital bed.

I get up and begin preparing breakfast anyway. Not for me but for Mom. She hasn't been eating. Perhaps if I bring her one of her favorites—a soft boiled egg with butter and pepper and salt—she'll eat a little.

Just as the water begins to simmer, the phone rings. It's the doctor on duty for the weekend. A stranger to me. He admits he was surprised when he noted there was still a CODE on Mom's chart. He wonders if I really want it to remain. There's compassion in his voice. I am upset by the oversight. We both agree, when the time comes, any attempt at resuscitation would only be cruel. Filled with gratitude for his caring I unhesitatingly give him permission to remove the CODE.

I continue preparation to leave for the hospital. Along with the cooked egg, I take a few necessities. From now on I am determined I won't leave Mom's bedside. No more sleep. Tonight God and I will keep watch.

⁂   ⁂   ⁂

C l o s u r e

Unannounced, at midnight, our friend arrives carrying doughnuts and hot coffee. She has driven in from her campsite to be with us. I am very grateful for her company.

Not wanting to exclude Mom who is unable to drink from a cup, we attempt to share our coffee with her by soaking her mouth sponge. The snack completed, our friend retreats to an unobtrusive chair in the corner where she maintains her silent vigil.

Shadows loom large in the soft light cast from the towel-covered desk lamp borrowed from the nurses' station.

Past grief experiences have taught me the importance of such a night as this. Between snatches of favorite hymns and comforting Bible passages, I tell Mom what a wonderful mother she has been. I remind her of the dream she once had in which God told her that when she was ready to die she had only to knock and the door would be opened. She was promised that under the darkness she would find the Everlasting Arms. Most importantly, I am able to tell her I am ready to have her leave, I will miss her but she doesn't have to worry, I will be fine.

Morning dawns.

✳   ✳   ✳

Her Parting Gift

Quietly, peacefully, at ninety-two, she left us. Her bright spirit gently being released as her breathing softened and finally stopped. This woman who, numerous times had successfully fought to live against all medical odds, now went without a trace of struggle.

We tenderly stroked and kissed her as she made her transition.

"Dear, dear Mom," my husband murmured, tears streaming down his face.

I found myself raising the bed clothes, wanting to take one more look at her pudgy little toes. Toes I had washed and covered so often. Every inch of her precious.

I had always known I loved her. When she was alive, however, I could never be completely sure this sense of love didn't emanate from all she was able to do for me or, in the later years, from my great dread of losing her. Now I knew. Without question the love I was feeling so deeply was unconditional. Gradually, spreading like a warm glow, came the realization that I, too, was lovable simply in my being. I didn't need to, nor could I ever, earn such lovability.

And today, as I write this final page, I want to pass on Mom's parting gift to you. I want you to know beyond a doubt that, without changing one aspect of yourself, you too, are lovable. You are lovable right here, right now and forever.

＊　＊　＊

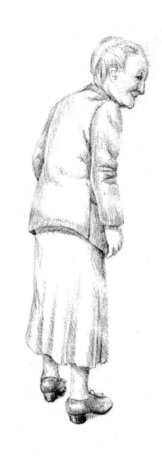

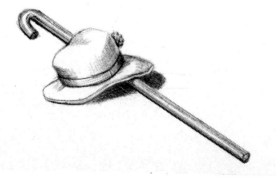

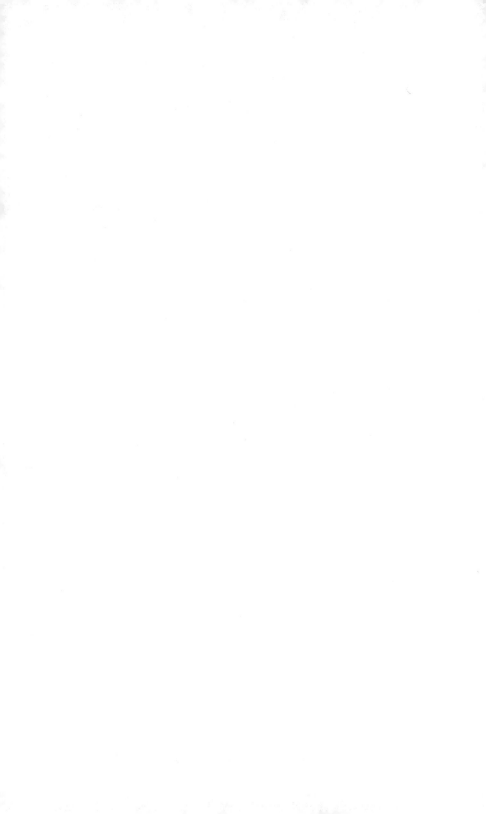